Workout Log

Name: _______________________________

Start Date: _______________________________

End Date: _______________________________

Always ensure that you consult your physician before beginning any exercise regimen.

Date: _______________ Location: _______________________________________

Start Time: _____________________ End Time: _____________________

Previous Night's Sleep (hours): _________ Quality (1-10): _________

Today's Meals and Times Eaten: _______________________________

____

____

____

____

____

____

Exercises and Notes (Sets, Reps, Times, Completion/Failure)

____

____

____

____

____

____

____

____

____

Positives from This Workout: ____________________________________

____

Things to Improve / Next Time Goals: ____________________________

____

____

Date: _____________ Location: _________________________________

Start Time: ___________________ End Time: ___________________

Previous Night's Sleep (hours): _________ Quality (1-10): _________

Today's Meals and Times Eaten: _______________________________

____

____

____

____

____

Exercises and Notes (Sets, Reps, Times, Completion/Failure)

____

____

____

____

____

____

____

____

____

Positives from This Workout: _________________________________

____

____

Things to Improve / Next Time Goals: _________________________

____

____

Date: _______________ Location: ________________________________

Start Time: __________________ End Time: __________________

Previous Night's Sleep (hours): ________ Quality (1-10): _________

Today's Meals and Times Eaten: ________________________________

____

____

____

____

____

Exercises and Notes (Sets, Reps, Times, Completion/Failure)

____

____

____

____

____

____

____

____

Positives from This Workout: ________________________________

____

____

Things to Improve / Next Time Goals: _____________________________

____

____

Date: ________________ Location: _________________________________

Start Time: ___________________ End Time: ____________________

Previous Night's Sleep (hours): __________ Quality (1-10): __________

Today's Meals and Times Eaten: _______________________________

____

____

____

____

____

Exercises and Notes (Sets, Reps, Times, Completion/Failure)

____

____

____

____

____

____

____

____

____

Positives from This Workout: ________________________________

____

____

Things to Improve / Next Time Goals: _________________________

____

____

Date: _______________ Location: _________________________________

Start Time: _________________ End Time: _________________

Previous Night's Sleep (hours): _________ Quality (1-10): _________

Today's Meals and Times Eaten: _____________________________

____

____

____

____

____

Exercises and Notes (Sets, Reps, Times, Completion/Failure)

____

____

____

____

____

____

____

____

Positives from This Workout: ___________________________________

____

Things to Improve / Next Time Goals: ____________________________

____

Date: _______________ Location: ___________________________________

Start Time: __________________ End Time: __________________

Previous Night's Sleep (hours): _________ Quality (1-10): __________

Today's Meals and Times Eaten: ___________________________________

____

____

____

____

____

Exercises and Notes (Sets, Reps, Times, Completion/Failure)

____

____

____

____

____

____

____

____

Positives from This Workout: ___________________________________

____

____

Things to Improve / Next Time Goals: ___________________________

____

____

Date: _______________ Location: _________________________________

Start Time: _____________________ End Time: ___________________________

Previous Night's Sleep (hours): _________ Quality (1-10): __________

Today's Meals and Times Eaten: _________________________________

____

____

____

____

____

Exercises and Notes (Sets, Reps, Times, Completion/Failure)

____

____

____

____

____

____

____

____

____

Positives from This Workout: _________________________________

____

Things to Improve / Next Time Goals: ___________________________

____

____

Date: _______________   Location: _________________________________

Start Time: ____________________   End Time: ___________________

Previous Night's Sleep (hours): __________ Quality (1-10): __________

Today's Meals and Times Eaten: ______________________________

____

____

____

____

____

Exercises and Notes (Sets, Reps, Times, Completion/Failure)

____

____

____

____

____

____

____

____

Positives from This Workout: __________________________________

____

____

Things to Improve / Next Time Goals: ____________________________

____

____

Date: _______________ Location: _________________________________

Start Time: _________________ End Time: _________________

Previous Night's Sleep (hours): _________ Quality (1-10): _________

Today's Meals and Times Eaten: _______________________________

____

____

____

____

____

Exercises and Notes (Sets, Reps, Times, Completion/Failure)

____

____

____

____

____

____

____

____

Positives from This Workout: _____________________________

____

Things to Improve / Next Time Goals: _____________________

____

Date: ______________ Location: _________________________________

Start Time: ___________________ End Time: ___________________

Previous Night's Sleep (hours): _________ Quality (1-10): _________

Today's Meals and Times Eaten: ____________________________

____

____

____

____

____

Exercises and Notes (Sets, Reps, Times, Completion/Failure)

____

____

____

____

____

____

____

____

____

Positives from This Workout: ______________________________

____

Things to Improve / Next Time Goals: ______________________

____

____

Date: _____________ **Location:** ________________________

Start Time: _______________ **End Time:** ________________

Previous Night's Sleep (hours): _________ **Quality (1-10):** _________

Today's Meals and Times Eaten: ________________________

____

____

____

____

____

Exercises and Notes (Sets, Reps, Times, Completion/Failure)

____

____

____

____

____

____

____

____

Positives from This Workout: ________________________

____

Things to Improve / Next Time Goals: ________________

____

____

Date: _______________ Location: _________________________________

Start Time: ___________________ End Time: __________________

Previous Night's Sleep (hours): _________ Quality (1-10): _________

Today's Meals and Times Eaten: _______________________________

____

____

____

____

____

____

Exercises and Notes (Sets, Reps, Times, Completion/Failure)

____

____

____

____

____

____

____

____

____

Positives from This Workout: ___________________________________

____

Things to Improve / Next Time Goals: ___________________________

____

____

Date: _______________ Location: _______________________________________

Start Time: _____________________ End Time: ______________________________

Previous Night's Sleep (hours): ________ Quality (1-10): _________

Today's Meals and Times Eaten: ____________________________________

____

____

____

____

____

Exercises and Notes (Sets, Reps, Times, Completion/Failure)

____

____

____

____

____

____

____

____

Positives from This Workout: _____________________________________

____

Things to Improve / Next Time Goals: _____________________________

____

____

Date: _____________ Location: _______________________________

Start Time: _________________ End Time: _________________

Previous Night's Sleep (hours): ________ Quality (1-10): ________

Today's Meals and Times Eaten: _______________________________

____

____

____

____

____

Exercises and Notes (Sets, Reps, Times, Completion/Failure)

____

____

____

____

____

____

____

____

____

Positives from This Workout: _______________________________

____

Things to Improve / Next Time Goals: _______________________

____

____

Date: _______________ Location: _______________________________

Start Time: __________________ End Time: ___________________

Previous Night's Sleep (hours): _________ Quality (1-10): _________

Today's Meals and Times Eaten: ___________________________________

____

____

____

____

____

Exercises and Notes (Sets, Reps, Times, Completion/Failure)

____

____

____

____

____

____

____

____

Positives from This Workout: _____________________________________

____

Things to Improve / Next Time Goals: ______________________________

____

____

Date: ________________ Location: _________________________________

Start Time: __________________ End Time: ____________________

Previous Night's Sleep (hours): _________ Quality (1-10): _________

Today's Meals and Times Eaten: _______________________________

____

____

____

____

____

Exercises and Notes (Sets, Reps, Times, Completion/Failure)

____

____

____

____

____

____

____

____

Positives from This Workout: _________________________________

____

Things to Improve / Next Time Goals: _________________________

____

____

Date: _____________ Location: _______________________________

Start Time: _______________ End Time: _______________

Previous Night's Sleep (hours): _________ Quality (1-10): _________

Today's Meals and Times Eaten: _______________________

____

____

____

____

____

Exercises and Notes (Sets, Reps, Times, Completion/Failure)

____

____

____

____

____

____

____

____

Positives from This Workout: ___________________________

____

Things to Improve / Next Time Goals: ___________________

____

____

Date: _______________ Location: ______________________________________

Start Time: __________________ End Time: __________________

Previous Night's Sleep (hours): _________ Quality (1-10): _________

Today's Meals and Times Eaten: _____________________________

____

____

____

____

____

____

Exercises and Notes (Sets, Reps, Times, Completion/Failure)

____

____

____

____

____

____

____

____

____

Positives from This Workout: ________________________________

____

Things to Improve / Next Time Goals: ________________________

____

Date: _______________ Location: _______________________________

Start Time: _____________________ End Time: ___________________

Previous Night's Sleep (hours): _________ Quality (1-10): _________

Today's Meals and Times Eaten: _________________________________

____

____

____

____

____

Exercises and Notes (Sets, Reps, Times, Completion/Failure)

____

____

____

____

____

____

____

____

Positives from This Workout: ___________________________________

____

Things to Improve / Next Time Goals: ____________________________

____

____

Date: ________________ Location: ______________________________________

Start Time: ____________________ End Time: ____________________

Previous Night's Sleep (hours): __________ Quality (1-10): __________

Today's Meals and Times Eaten: ______________________________

____

____

____

____

____

Exercises and Notes (Sets, Reps, Times, Completion/Failure)

____

____

____

____

____

____

____

____

____

Positives from This Workout: ______________________________

____

____

Things to Improve / Next Time Goals: ______________________

____

____

Date: ______________ Location: ___________________________________

Start Time: _________________ End Time: ____________________

Previous Night's Sleep (hours): _______ Quality (1-10): _________

Today's Meals and Times Eaten: _______________________________

____

____

____

____

____

Exercises and Notes (Sets, Reps, Times, Completion/Failure)

____

____

____

____

____

____

____

____

Positives from This Workout: _________________________________

____

Things to Improve / Next Time Goals: __________________________

____

Date: _____________ Location: _________________________________

Start Time: _________________ End Time: ___________________

Previous Night's Sleep (hours): _________ Quality (1-10): _________

Today's Meals and Times Eaten: ____________________________

____

____

____

____

____

Exercises and Notes (Sets, Reps, Times, Completion/Failure)

____

____

____

____

____

____

____

____

Positives from This Workout: _____________________________

____

____

Things to Improve / Next Time Goals: _____________________

____

____

Date: _______________ Location: _________________________________

Start Time: _________________ End Time: _____________________

Previous Night's Sleep (hours): _________ Quality (1-10): _________

Today's Meals and Times Eaten: _______________________________

____

____

____

____

____

____

Exercises and Notes (Sets, Reps, Times, Completion/Failure)

____

____

____

____

____

____

____

____

____

Positives from This Workout: _________________________________

____

____

Things to Improve / Next Time Goals: _________________________

____

____

Date: _______________ Location: ____

Start Time: ____________________ End Time: ____________________

Previous Night's Sleep (hours): _________ Quality (1-10): __________

Today's Meals and Times Eaten: _______________________________

____

____

____

____

____

Exercises and Notes (Sets, Reps, Times, Completion/Failure)

____

____

____

____

____

____

____

____

Positives from This Workout: _________________________________

____

Things to Improve / Next Time Goals: _________________________

____

____

Date: _______________ Location: ___________________________

Start Time: _________________ End Time: _________________

Previous Night's Sleep (hours): _______ Quality (1-10): _______

Today's Meals and Times Eaten: _______________________________

____

____

____

____

____

Exercises and Notes (Sets, Reps, Times, Completion/Failure)

____

____

____

____

____

____

____

____

Positives from This Workout: _______________________________

____

Things to Improve / Next Time Goals: _______________________

____

Date: _______________ Location: _________________________________

Start Time: _________________ End Time: _________________

Previous Night's Sleep (hours): _________ Quality (1-10): _________

Today's Meals and Times Eaten: _________________________________

____

____

____

____

____

Exercises and Notes (Sets, Reps, Times, Completion/Failure)

____

____

____

____

____

____

____

____

____

Positives from This Workout: _____________________________________

____

Things to Improve / Next Time Goals: _____________________________

____

____

Date: _______________ Location: _________________________________

Start Time: _________________ End Time: _________________

Previous Night's Sleep (hours): _________ Quality (1-10): _________

Today's Meals and Times Eaten:_________________________________

____

____

____

____

____

____

Exercises and Notes (Sets, Reps, Times, Completion/Failure)

____

____

____

____

____

____

____

____

____

Positives from This Workout: ___________________________________

____

____

Things to Improve / Next Time Goals:____________________________

____

____

Date: _______________ Location: _______________________________________

Start Time: ___________________ End Time: ____________________

Previous Night's Sleep (hours): _________ Quality (1-10): _________

Today's Meals and Times Eaten: ____________________________________

____

____

____

____

____

Exercises and Notes (Sets, Reps, Times, Completion/Failure)

____

____

____

____

____

____

____

____

____

Positives from This Workout: _____________________________________

____

Things to Improve / Next Time Goals: ______________________________

____

____

Date: _______________ Location: _________________________________

Start Time: _________________ End Time: _________________

Previous Night's Sleep (hours): ________ Quality (1-10): ________

Today's Meals and Times Eaten: _______________________________

____

____

____

____

____

Exercises and Notes (Sets, Reps, Times, Completion/Failure)

____

____

____

____

____

____

____

____

Positives from This Workout: _________________________________

____

Things to Improve / Next Time Goals: _________________________

____

____

Date: _______________ Location: ________________________________

Start Time: __________________ End Time: ___________________

Previous Night's Sleep (hours): _________ Quality (1-10): _________

Today's Meals and Times Eaten: _______________________________

____

____

____

____

____

____

Exercises and Notes (Sets, Reps, Times, Completion/Failure)

____

____

____

____

____

____

____

____

____

Positives from This Workout: ___________________________________

____

____

Things to Improve / Next Time Goals: ___________________________

____

____

Date: _______________ Location: _________________________________

Start Time: ___________________ End Time: __________________

Previous Night's Sleep (hours): _________ Quality (1-10): _________

Today's Meals and Times Eaten: _______________________________

____

____

____

____

____

Exercises and Notes (Sets, Reps, Times, Completion/Failure)

____

____

____

____

____

____

____

____

____

Positives from This Workout: _________________________________

____

Things to Improve / Next Time Goals: _________________________

____

____

Date: _____________ Location: _________________________________

Start Time: _________________ End Time: _________________

Previous Night's Sleep (hours): _________ Quality (1-10): _________

Today's Meals and Times Eaten: _______________________________

____

____

____

____

____

Exercises and Notes (Sets, Reps, Times, Completion/Failure)

____

____

____

____

____

____

____

____

Positives from This Workout: _________________________________

____

Things to Improve / Next Time Goals: _________________________

____

____

Date: _______________ Location: ______________________________

Start Time: _______________ End Time: _______________________

Previous Night's Sleep (hours): _________ Quality (1-10): _________

Today's Meals and Times Eaten: ________________________________

____

____

____

____

____

____

Exercises and Notes (Sets, Reps, Times, Completion/Failure)

____

____

____

____

____

____

____

____

____

Positives from This Workout: __________________________________

____

____

Things to Improve / Next Time Goals: ___________________________

____

____

Date: _______________ Location: _________________________________

Start Time: __________________ End Time: __________________

Previous Night's Sleep (hours): _________ Quality (1-10): _________

Today's Meals and Times Eaten: _________________________________

____

____

____

____

____

Exercises and Notes (Sets, Reps, Times, Completion/Failure)

____

____

____

____

____

____

____

____

Positives from This Workout: ____________________________________

____

Things to Improve / Next Time Goals: ____________________________

____

____

Date: _______________ Location: _________________________________

Start Time: _________________ End Time: _________________________

Previous Night's Sleep (hours): _________ Quality (1-10): _________

Today's Meals and Times Eaten: _________________________________

____

____

____

____

____

Exercises and Notes (Sets, Reps, Times, Completion/Failure)

____

____

____

____

____

____

____

____

Positives from This Workout: _____________________________________

____

Things to Improve / Next Time Goals: _____________________________

____

____

Date: _______________ Location: ____________________________________

Start Time: __________________ End Time: ___________________

Previous Night's Sleep (hours): _________ Quality (1-10): _________

Today's Meals and Times Eaten: _____________________________

____

____

____

____

____

____

Exercises and Notes (Sets, Reps, Times, Completion/Failure)

____

____

____

____

____

____

____

____

____

____

Positives from This Workout: _________________________________

____

____

Things to Improve / Next Time Goals: _________________________

____

____

Date: _______________ Location: ____________________________________

Start Time: _____________________ End Time: ______________________

Previous Night's Sleep (hours): __________ Quality (1-10): _________

Today's Meals and Times Eaten: ___________________________________

____

____

____

____

____

Exercises and Notes (Sets, Reps, Times, Completion/Failure)

____

____

____

____

____

____

____

____

Positives from This Workout: _____________________________________

____

Things to Improve / Next Time Goals: ______________________________

____

____

Date: _______________ Location: _________________________________

Start Time: _____________________ End Time: _____________________

Previous Night's Sleep (hours): _________ Quality (1-10): _________

Today's Meals and Times Eaten: _________________________________

____

____

____

____

____

Exercises and Notes (Sets, Reps, Times, Completion/Failure)

____

____

____

____

____

____

____

____

____

Positives from This Workout: _________________________________

____

____

Things to Improve / Next Time Goals: _____________________________

____

____

Date: _______________ Location: _________________________________

Start Time: _________________ End Time: _____________________

Previous Night's Sleep (hours): _________ Quality (1-10): __________

Today's Meals and Times Eaten: _______________________________

____

____

____

____

____

Exercises and Notes (Sets, Reps, Times, Completion/Failure)

____

____

____

____

____

____

____

____

____

Positives from This Workout: _________________________________

____

Things to Improve / Next Time Goals: __________________________

____

Date: _______________ Location: ________________________________

Start Time: __________________ End Time: __________________

Previous Night's Sleep (hours): _________ Quality (1-10): _________

Today's Meals and Times Eaten: ________________________________

____

____

____

____

____

Exercises and Notes (Sets, Reps, Times, Completion/Failure)

____

____

____

____

____

____

____

____

____

Positives from This Workout: ________________________________

____

____

Things to Improve / Next Time Goals: ________________________

____

____

Date: _______________ Location: ___________________________

Start Time: __________________ End Time: ___________________

Previous Night's Sleep (hours): _________ Quality (1-10): _________

Today's Meals and Times Eaten: ______________________________

____

____

____

____

____

____

Exercises and Notes (Sets, Reps, Times, Completion/Failure)

____

____

____

____

____

____

____

____

____

Positives from This Workout: _________________________________

____

____

Things to Improve / Next Time Goals: ___________________________

____

____

Date: _____________ Location: _________________________________

Start Time: _________________ End Time: __________________

Previous Night's Sleep (hours): ________ Quality (1-10): ________

Today's Meals and Times Eaten: ____________________________

____

____

____

____

____

Exercises and Notes (Sets, Reps, Times, Completion/Failure)

____

____

____

____

____

____

____

____

____

Positives from This Workout: _______________________________

____

Things to Improve / Next Time Goals: ________________________

____

____

Date: _______________ Location: _________________________________

Start Time: _________________ End Time: __________________

Previous Night's Sleep (hours): ________ Quality (1-10): _________

Today's Meals and Times Eaten: ________________________________

____

____

____

____

____

Exercises and Notes (Sets, Reps, Times, Completion/Failure)

____

____

____

____

____

____

____

____

Positives from This Workout: ___________________________________

____

Things to Improve / Next Time Goals: ___________________________

____

Date: _____________ Location: _________________________________

Start Time: _________________ End Time: _________________

Previous Night's Sleep (hours): ________ Quality (1-10): ________

Today's Meals and Times Eaten: _______________________________

____

____

____

____

____

Exercises and Notes (Sets, Reps, Times, Completion/Failure)

____

____

____

____

____

____

____

____

____

Positives from This Workout: _________________________________

____

____

Things to Improve / Next Time Goals: __________________________

____

____

Date: _______________ Location: ________________________________

Start Time: ________________ End Time: ___________________

Previous Night's Sleep (hours): ________ Quality (1-10): _________

Today's Meals and Times Eaten: ______________________________

____

____

____

____

____

Exercises and Notes (Sets, Reps, Times, Completion/Failure)

____

____

____

____

____

____

____

____

____

Positives from This Workout: _________________________________

____

____

Things to Improve / Next Time Goals: __________________________

____

____

Date: _______________ Location: _______________________________________

Start Time: __________________ End Time: ___________________

Previous Night's Sleep (hours): _________ Quality (1-10): _________

Today's Meals and Times Eaten: ________________________________

____

____

____

____

____

Exercises and Notes (Sets, Reps, Times, Completion/Failure)

____

____

____

____

____

____

____

____

Positives from This Workout: __________________________________

____

Things to Improve / Next Time Goals: ___________________________

____

____

Date: _______________ Location: _________________________________

Start Time: _________________ End Time: _________________

Previous Night's Sleep (hours): _________ Quality (1-10): _________

Today's Meals and Times Eaten: _________________________________

____

____

____

____

____

Exercises and Notes (Sets, Reps, Times, Completion/Failure)

____

____

____

____

____

____

____

____

Positives from This Workout: _____________________________________

____

Things to Improve / Next Time Goals: _____________________________

____

____

Date: _______________ Location: _______________________________________

Start Time: ___________________ End Time: ____________________

Previous Night's Sleep (hours): _________ Quality (1-10): _________

Today's Meals and Times Eaten: _______________________________

____

____

____

____

____

Exercises and Notes (Sets, Reps, Times, Completion/Failure)

____

____

____

____

____

____

____

____

____

Positives from This Workout: __________________________________

____

Things to Improve / Next Time Goals: __________________________

____

____

Date: ________________   Location: ____________________________________

Start Time: _____________________   End Time: ____________________

Previous Night's Sleep (hours): __________ Quality (1-10): __________

Today's Meals and Times Eaten: ________________________________

____

____

____

____

____

Exercises and Notes (Sets, Reps, Times, Completion/Failure)

____

____

____

____

____

____

____

____

Positives from This Workout: ___________________________________

____

Things to Improve / Next Time Goals: ___________________________

____

Date: _______________ Location: _________________________________

Start Time: __________________ End Time: _________________

Previous Night's Sleep (hours): _________ Quality (1-10): _________

Today's Meals and Times Eaten: _____________________________

____

____

____

____

____

Exercises and Notes (Sets, Reps, Times, Completion/Failure)

____

____

____

____

____

____

____

____

____

Positives from This Workout: _______________________________

____

Things to Improve / Next Time Goals: _______________________

____

____

Date: ________________ Location: ______________________________

Start Time: ____________________ End Time: ___________________

Previous Night's Sleep (hours): _________ Quality (1-10): _________

Today's Meals and Times Eaten: ___________________________

____

____

____

____

____

Exercises and Notes (Sets, Reps, Times, Completion/Failure)

____

____

____

____

____

____

____

____

Positives from This Workout: _______________________________

____

Things to Improve / Next Time Goals: _______________________

____

____

Date: _______________ Location: ____________________________________

Start Time: ___________________ End Time: _________________________

Previous Night's Sleep (hours): _________ Quality (1-10): _________

Today's Meals and Times Eaten: _____________________________________

____

____

____

____

____

Exercises and Notes (Sets, Reps, Times, Completion/Failure)

____

____

____

____

____

____

____

____

Positives from This Workout: _______________________________________

____

Things to Improve / Next Time Goals: _______________________________

____

____

Date: _______________ Location: ___________________________________

Start Time: ___________________ End Time: __________________

Previous Night's Sleep (hours): _________ Quality (1-10): _________

Today's Meals and Times Eaten: _______________________________

____

____

____

____

____

Exercises and Notes (Sets, Reps, Times, Completion/Failure)

____

____

____

____

____

____

____

____

Positives from This Workout: _________________________________

____

Things to Improve / Next Time Goals: __________________________

____

Date: _____________ Location: ________________________________

Start Time: _________________ End Time: _________________

Previous Night's Sleep (hours): ________ Quality (1-10): ________

Today's Meals and Times Eaten: ______________________________

____

____

____

____

____

Exercises and Notes (Sets, Reps, Times, Completion/Failure)

____

____

____

____

____

____

____

____

____

Positives from This Workout: _________________________________

____

Things to Improve / Next Time Goals: _________________________

____

Date: _______________ Location: _________________________________

Start Time: _________________ End Time: _____________________

Previous Night's Sleep (hours): _________ Quality (1-10): _________

Today's Meals and Times Eaten: _________________________________

____

____

____

____

____

Exercises and Notes (Sets, Reps, Times, Completion/Failure)

____

____

____

____

____

____

____

____

Positives from This Workout: ____________________________________

____

Things to Improve / Next Time Goals: ____________________________

____

____

Date: _______________ Location: _________________________________

Start Time: _________________ End Time: _________________

Previous Night's Sleep (hours): _________ Quality (1-10): _________

Today's Meals and Times Eaten: _________________________________

____

____

____

____

____

Exercises and Notes (Sets, Reps, Times, Completion/Failure)

____

____

____

____

____

____

____

____

Positives from This Workout: _________________________________

____

____

Things to Improve / Next Time Goals: _________________________

____

____

Date: _______________ Location: _________________________________

Start Time: _________________ End Time: _________________________

Previous Night's Sleep (hours): _________ Quality (1-10): _________

Today's Meals and Times Eaten: ___________________________________

____

____

____

____

____

Exercises and Notes (Sets, Reps, Times, Completion/Failure)

____

____

____

____

____

____

____

____

Positives from This Workout: _____________________________________

____

____

Things to Improve / Next Time Goals: ______________________________

____

____

Date: _____________ **Location:** _______________________________

Start Time: _________________ **End Time:** _________________

Previous Night's Sleep (hours): ________ **Quality (1-10):** ________

Today's Meals and Times Eaten: ______________________________

____

____

____

____

____

Exercises and Notes (Sets, Reps, Times, Completion/Failure)

____

____

____

____

____

____

____

____

Positives from This Workout: ________________________________

____

Things to Improve / Next Time Goals: _________________________

____

____

Date: _____________ Location: _______________________________

Start Time: _________________ End Time: _______________

Previous Night's Sleep (hours): _______ Quality (1-10): ________

Today's Meals and Times Eaten: _______________________________

____

____

____

____

____

Exercises and Notes (Sets, Reps, Times, Completion/Failure)

____

____

____

____

____

____

____

____

Positives from This Workout: _______________________________

____

Things to Improve / Next Time Goals: _______________________

____

Date: _______________ Location: _________________________________

Start Time: __________________ End Time: ____________________

Previous Night's Sleep (hours): _________ Quality (1-10): _________

Today's Meals and Times Eaten: ________________________________

____

____

____

____

____

Exercises and Notes (Sets, Reps, Times, Completion/Failure)

____

____

____

____

____

____

____

____

____

Positives from This Workout: ___________________________________

____

Things to Improve / Next Time Goals: ____________________________

____

Date: _______________ Location: _________________________________

Start Time: _________________ End Time: _____________________

Previous Night's Sleep (hours): _________ Quality (1-10): _________

Today's Meals and Times Eaten: _________________________________

____

____

____

____

____

Exercises and Notes (Sets, Reps, Times, Completion/Failure)

____

____

____

____

____

____

____

____

____

Positives from This Workout: ___________________________________

____

____

Things to Improve / Next Time Goals: ___________________________

____

____

Date: _______________ Location: ___________________________________

Start Time: __________________ End Time: ___________________

Previous Night's Sleep (hours): _________ Quality (1-10): _________

Today's Meals and Times Eaten: _______________________________

____

____

____

____

____

Exercises and Notes (Sets, Reps, Times, Completion/Failure)

____

____

____

____

____

____

____

____

____

Positives from This Workout: ___________________________________

____

____

Things to Improve / Next Time Goals: ___________________________

____

____

Date: _______________ Location: _________________________________

Start Time: _________________ End Time: _______________________

Previous Night's Sleep (hours): ________ Quality (1-10): _________

Today's Meals and Times Eaten: _________________________________

____

____

____

____

____

____

Exercises and Notes (Sets, Reps, Times, Completion/Failure)

____

____

____

____

____

____

____

____

Positives from This Workout: ___________________________________

____

Things to Improve / Next Time Goals: ____________________________

____

____

Date: _______________ Location: _________________________________

Start Time: _____________________ End Time: ____________________

Previous Night's Sleep (hours): _________ Quality (1-10): _________

Today's Meals and Times Eaten: _______________________________

____

____

____

____

____

Exercises and Notes (Sets, Reps, Times, Completion/Failure)

____

____

____

____

____

____

____

____

____

Positives from This Workout: _________________________________

____

Things to Improve / Next Time Goals: __________________________

____

____

Date: _______________ Location: _________________________________

Start Time: _____________________ End Time: ____________________

Previous Night's Sleep (hours): _________ Quality (1-10): _________

Today's Meals and Times Eaten: _________________________________

____

____

____

____

____

Exercises and Notes (Sets, Reps, Times, Completion/Failure)

____

____

____

____

____

____

____

____

____

Positives from This Workout: ____________________________________

____

Things to Improve / Next Time Goals: ____________________________

____

____

Date: _______________ Location: ___________________________________

Start Time: _____________________ End Time: ____________________

Previous Night's Sleep (hours): _________ Quality (1-10): _________

Today's Meals and Times Eaten: ______________________________

____

____

____

____

____

Exercises and Notes (Sets, Reps, Times, Completion/Failure)

____

____

____

____

____

____

____

____

____

Positives from This Workout: ________________________________

____

Things to Improve / Next Time Goals: _________________________

____

____

Date: ________________ Location: _________________________________

Start Time: __________________ End Time: __________________

Previous Night's Sleep (hours): ________ Quality (1-10): _________

Today's Meals and Times Eaten: _________________________________

____

____

____

____

____

Exercises and Notes (Sets, Reps, Times, Completion/Failure)

____

____

____

____

____

____

____

____

Positives from This Workout: _________________________________

____

Things to Improve / Next Time Goals: ___________________________

____

____

Date: _______________ Location: _________________________________

Start Time: __________________ End Time: _________________

Previous Night's Sleep (hours): _________ Quality (1-10): _________

Today's Meals and Times Eaten: _______________________________

____

____

____

____

____

Exercises and Notes (Sets, Reps, Times, Completion/Failure)

____

____

____

____

____

____

____

____

Positives from This Workout: ________________________________

____

Things to Improve / Next Time Goals: _________________________

____

Date: _______________ Location: _________________________________

Start Time: _________________ End Time: _____________________

Previous Night's Sleep (hours): _________ Quality (1-10): _________

Today's Meals and Times Eaten: _____________________________

____

____

____

____

____

Exercises and Notes (Sets, Reps, Times, Completion/Failure)

____

____

____

____

____

____

____

____

Positives from This Workout: _______________________________

____

Things to Improve / Next Time Goals: _______________________

____

Date: ________________   Location: ________________________________

Start Time: __________________   End Time: __________________

Previous Night's Sleep (hours): ________ Quality (1-10): ________

Today's Meals and Times Eaten: ______________________________

____

____

____

____

____

Exercises and Notes (Sets, Reps, Times, Completion/Failure)

____

____

____

____

____

____

____

____

____

Positives from This Workout: ______________________________

____

____

Things to Improve / Next Time Goals: ______________________

____

____

Date: _______________ **Location:** _________________________________

Start Time: ___________________ **End Time:** ___________________

Previous Night's Sleep (hours): _________ **Quality (1-10):** _________

Today's Meals and Times Eaten: _______________________________

____

____

____

____

____

Exercises and Notes (Sets, Reps, Times, Completion/Failure)

____

____

____

____

____

____

____

____

Positives from This Workout: _________________________________

____

Things to Improve / Next Time Goals: _________________________

____

____

Date: _______________ Location: _________________________________

Start Time: __________________ End Time: ___________________

Previous Night's Sleep (hours): _________ Quality (1-10): _________

Today's Meals and Times Eaten: _______________________________

____

____

____

____

____

Exercises and Notes (Sets, Reps, Times, Completion/Failure)

____

____

____

____

____

____

____

____

Positives from This Workout: _________________________________

____

Things to Improve / Next Time Goals: ___________________________

____

Date: _____________ Location: _______________________________

Start Time: _________________ End Time: ___________________

Previous Night's Sleep (hours): ________ Quality (1-10): ________

Today's Meals and Times Eaten: _______________________________

____

____

____

____

____

Exercises and Notes (Sets, Reps, Times, Completion/Failure)

____

____

____

____

____

____

____

____

Positives from This Workout: _________________________________

____

Things to Improve / Next Time Goals: _________________________

____

____

Date: _______________ Location: _________________________________

Start Time: ___________________ End Time: ____________________

Previous Night's Sleep (hours): _________ Quality (1-10): _________

Today's Meals and Times Eaten: ___________________________

____

____

____

____

____

Exercises and Notes (Sets, Reps, Times, Completion/Failure)

____

____

____

____

____

____

____

____

Positives from This Workout: ________________________________

____

____

Things to Improve / Next Time Goals: _________________________

____

____

Date: _______________ Location: _________________________________

Start Time: _________________ End Time: ___________________

Previous Night's Sleep (hours): _________ Quality (1-10): _________

Today's Meals and Times Eaten: _________________________________

____

____

____

____

____

Exercises and Notes (Sets, Reps, Times, Completion/Failure)

____

____

____

____

____

____

____

____

Positives from This Workout: ____________________________________

____

Things to Improve / Next Time Goals: ____________________________

____

____

Date: _______________ Location: ___________________________________

Start Time: __________________ End Time: ___________________

Previous Night's Sleep (hours): _________ Quality (1-10): _________

Today's Meals and Times Eaten: _______________________________

____

____

____

____

____

Exercises and Notes (Sets, Reps, Times, Completion/Failure)

____

____

____

____

____

____

____

____

____

Positives from This Workout: _________________________________

____

____

Things to Improve / Next Time Goals: _________________________

____

____

Date: _______________ Location: ___________________________________

Start Time: __________________ End Time: __________________

Previous Night's Sleep (hours): _________ Quality (1-10): _________

Today's Meals and Times Eaten: _________________________________

____

____

____

____

____

Exercises and Notes (Sets, Reps, Times, Completion/Failure)

____

____

____

____

____

____

____

____

Positives from This Workout: ________________________________

____

____

Things to Improve / Next Time Goals: _________________________

____

____

Date: _______________ Location: _________________________________

Start Time: _________________ End Time: ___________________

Previous Night's Sleep (hours): ________ Quality (1-10): ________

Today's Meals and Times Eaten: _______________________________

____

____

____

____

____

Exercises and Notes (Sets, Reps, Times, Completion/Failure)

____

____

____

____

____

____

____

____

____

Positives from This Workout: _________________________________

____

Things to Improve / Next Time Goals: ___________________________

____

____

Date: _______________ Location: _________________________________

Start Time: __________________ End Time: ___________________

Previous Night's Sleep (hours): _________ Quality (1-10): __________

Today's Meals and Times Eaten: ________________________________

____

____

____

____

____

Exercises and Notes (Sets, Reps, Times, Completion/Failure)

____

____

____

____

____

____

____

____

Positives from This Workout: _________________________________

____

____

Things to Improve / Next Time Goals: __________________________

____

____

Date: _____________ Location: _________________________________

Start Time: _________________ End Time: ___________________

Previous Night's Sleep (hours): _________ Quality (1-10): _________

Today's Meals and Times Eaten: ___________________________

____

____

____

____

____

Exercises and Notes (Sets, Reps, Times, Completion/Failure)

____

____

____

____

____

____

____

____

____

Positives from This Workout: _______________________________

____

____

Things to Improve / Next Time Goals: _____________________

____

____

Date: _______________ Location: ______________________________

Start Time: ________________ End Time: ___________________

Previous Night's Sleep (hours): _________ Quality (1-10): _________

Today's Meals and Times Eaten: ________________________________

____

____

____

____

____

Exercises and Notes (Sets, Reps, Times, Completion/Failure)

____

____

____

____

____

____

____

____

____

Positives from This Workout: __________________________________

____

Things to Improve / Next Time Goals: ___________________________

____

____

Date: ________________ Location: ___________________________________

Start Time: ____________________ End Time: ____________________

Previous Night's Sleep (hours): _________ Quality (1-10): _________

Today's Meals and Times Eaten: ___________________________________

____

____

____

____

____

Exercises and Notes (Sets, Reps, Times, Completion/Failure)

____

____

____

____

____

____

____

____

Positives from This Workout: ______________________________________

____

Things to Improve / Next Time Goals: ______________________________

____

____

Date: _______________ Location: ________________________________

Start Time: _________________ End Time: ___________________

Previous Night's Sleep (hours): _______ Quality (1-10): _________

Today's Meals and Times Eaten:________________________________

____

____

____

____

____

Exercises and Notes (Sets, Reps, Times, Completion/Failure)

____

____

____

____

____

____

____

____

Positives from This Workout: _________________________________

____

Things to Improve / Next Time Goals:__________________________

____

____

Date: _______________ Location: ___________________________________

Start Time: __________________ End Time: ___________________

Previous Night's Sleep (hours): _________ Quality (1-10): _________

Today's Meals and Times Eaten: ___________________________________

____

____

____

____

____

Exercises and Notes (Sets, Reps, Times, Completion/Failure)

____

____

____

____

____

____

____

____

____

Positives from This Workout: _____________________________________

____

Things to Improve / Next Time Goals: _____________________________

____

____

Date: _____________ Location: _______________________________

Start Time: _________________ End Time: _______________________

Previous Night's Sleep (hours): _________ Quality (1-10): _________

Today's Meals and Times Eaten: _______________________________

____

____

____

____

____

Exercises and Notes (Sets, Reps, Times, Completion/Failure)

____

____

____

____

____

____

____

____

____

Positives from This Workout: _________________________________

____

Things to Improve / Next Time Goals: _________________________

____

Date: _______________ Location: _________________________________

Start Time: __________________ End Time: ___________________

Previous Night's Sleep (hours): _________ Quality (1-10): _________

Today's Meals and Times Eaten: ________________________________

____

____

____

____

____

Exercises and Notes (Sets, Reps, Times, Completion/Failure)

____

____

____

____

____

____

____

____

____

Positives from This Workout: _________________________________

____

____

Things to Improve / Next Time Goals: _________________________

____

____

Date: _______________ Location: _______________________________

Start Time: _________________ End Time: _________________

Previous Night's Sleep (hours): ________ Quality (1-10): ________

Today's Meals and Times Eaten: _______________________________

____

____

____

____

____

Exercises and Notes (Sets, Reps, Times, Completion/Failure)

____

____

____

____

____

____

____

____

____

Positives from This Workout: _________________________________

____

____

Things to Improve / Next Time Goals: _________________________

____

____

Date: _______________ Location: _________________________________

Start Time: __________________ End Time: ___________________

Previous Night's Sleep (hours): _________ Quality (1-10): _________

Today's Meals and Times Eaten: _________________________________

____

____

____

____

____

____

Exercises and Notes (Sets, Reps, Times, Completion/Failure)

____

____

____

____

____

____

____

____

____

____

Positives from This Workout: ____________________________________

____

____

Things to Improve / Next Time Goals: ____________________________

____

____

Date: _______________ Location: _________________________________

Start Time: ___________________ End Time: __________________

Previous Night's Sleep (hours): _________ Quality (1-10): _________

Today's Meals and Times Eaten: _________________________________

____

____

____

____

____

Exercises and Notes (Sets, Reps, Times, Completion/Failure)

____

____

____

____

____

____

____

____

Positives from This Workout: ____________________________________

____

Things to Improve / Next Time Goals: ____________________________

____

____

Date: _______________ Location: _________________________________

Start Time: __________________ End Time: ___________________

Previous Night's Sleep (hours): _________ Quality (1-10): _________

Today's Meals and Times Eaten: _________________________________

____

____

____

____

____

Exercises and Notes (Sets, Reps, Times, Completion/Failure)

____

____

____

____

____

____

____

____

____

Positives from This Workout: ____________________________________

____

____

Things to Improve / Next Time Goals: ____________________________

____

____